For The Love Of NICU

For The Love Of NICU

Where the Heart Breaks
Open and Healing Begins

MELECIA HARRIOTT-MORANT

meleciaharriottmorant.com

Book Cover Design by Author, Melecia Harriott-Morant

Editing by Erica Zarrieff

Layout by Capture Your Brilliance LLC

Library of Congress Control Number (LCCN): 2026914587

ISBN Hardback: 979-8-9963643-9-8

ISBN Paperback: 979-8-9963643-7-4

ISBN eBook: 979-8-9963643-8-1

ISBN Audio Book: 979-8-9963643-6-7

Dedication

To the tiny fighters in the isolettes (incubators) and the giants standing beside them.

To the warriors who arrived early, fought harder, and redefined what it means to be resilient: you are not just survivors. You are the strongest among us, possessing courage that dwarfs the machines meant to save you.

To the parents standing in the trenches: I see the exhaustion in your bones and the courage in your quietest whispers. You have faced the impossible, navigated the ledge, and anchored your family when the world felt like it was spinning out of sync. May this book be the map you didn't know you needed, and the evidence reminding you that you are always the expert your child requires.

To the parents who carry their miracles in their hearts rather than their arms: this space belongs to you. Your journey has reached a sacred horizon. Your child's life is worthy, whole, and deeply valuable—it is a legacy of pure, unshakeable light.

For every mother and father who has lived a lifetime between the beeps of a monitor, the high alert ends here. You have fought the good fight with everything you had. May you find the grace to breathe, the space to heal, and the peace of knowing that your love is, was, and always will be, greater than the storm you know.

Contents

Foreword IX

Acknowledgements XI

Introduction 1

1. The Shock of the Unexpected 5
2. Life Inside the NICU 13
3. Coping with Emotional Overwhelm 23
4. Finding Your Role as a Parent 37
5. The NICU Rollercoaster 45
6. A Letter to the One Carrying a Miracle in Their Heart 55
7. Sustaining the Parent Behind the Miracle 61
8. Taking the Reigns 73

Epilogue: A Parent's Heart 81

Appendix A 83

Appendix B 85

Additional Resources from Melecia 89

Foreword

By Dr. Misael Mitch Rodriguez, MD

It is a privilege to write a few words in support of this remarkable book, For the Love of NICU, and its author, Nurse Melecia Harriott-Morant. I have known Ms. Harriott-Morant since she joined the Neonatal Intensive Care Unit (NICU) team at Atrium Health in February 2020.

During my 25 years as the *Medical Director* of the Neonatal Intensive Care Unit at the Beverly Knight Olsen Children's Hospital, I had the opportunity to work alongside countless dedicated professionals. Few embodied compassion, commitment, and advocacy for families as completely as Ms. Harriott-Morant.

As a Regional Perinatal Center, our neonatal unit cared for more than 750 admissions each year. We served infants and families during some of the most vulnerable and emotionally challenging moments of their lives. While neonatal medicine is grounded in science, technology, and highly specialized care, we learned repeatedly that families also need reassurance, understanding, practical guidance, and hope. *For the Love of NICU* speaks directly to those needs.

What makes this resource especially meaningful is that it was written by someone who has lived the NICU experience from the bedside every day. Ms. Harriott-Morant understands not only the medical complexities faced by premature and critically ill newborns, but also the fear, uncertainty, exhaustion, and resilience of parents navigating this journey. The wisdom contained in these pages comes from years of caring for infants while simultaneously supporting mothers, fathers, grandparents, and siblings through moments of crisis and celebration alike.

Throughout my career, I witnessed extraordinary advances in neonatal medicine that improved survival and outcomes for our smallest patients. Yet one truth remained constant: family-centered care is essential to healing. Parents are not simply visitors in the NICU—they are integral members of the care team. Providing them with knowledge, support, and confidence has lasting benefits for both the infant and the family. *For the Love of NICU* reflects that philosophy beautifully.

I am deeply grateful for the dedication and compassion Ms. Harriott-Morant has brought to our unit and to the many families whose lives have been touched by her work. I have no doubt that this resource will provide comfort, guidance, and encouragement to parents facing the challenges of a NICU hospitalization, while also serving as a valuable reference for caregivers and healthcare professionals in understanding the stressors that a NICU stay has on a family.

The families who enter a neonatal intensive care unit (NICU) begin a journey they never expected. My hope is that within these pages, they will find practical guidance, compassionate support, and the reassurance that they are not alone. May this resource provide the understanding, comfort, and courage they need, and help them recognize when it is time—it is ok to ask for help.

Dr. Misael Mitch Rodriguez, MD
Former Medical Director
Neonatal Intensive Care Unit
Beverly Knight Olsen Children's Hospital
Atrium Advocate Healthcare

Acknowledgements

I give all glory to God for planting this seed in my heart. A seed designed to help parents of the most vulnerable, yet resilient, warriors heal, find peace, and solace. This is more than a written work—it is a call to action, legacy, and hope.

To my spiritual support, you have carried me in prayer; your intercession gave me strength to continue when the emotional weight of this mission felt too great to carry.

To my husband, thank you for anchoring me with unwavering love and support. You understood the fire inside me, and you held my hand throughout the journey. I am honored to have you by my side.

To my family, you cheered for me the loudest when the room was quiet and stood with me when the world felt like it was falling apart.

To my children, you are my 'why.' I love you beyond measure and am blessed to be your mama. For you, I build a legacy you can one day be proud to call your own.

Introduction

Sometimes, the smallest lives are the ones that crack us wide open.

From the flutter of excitement of that first gentle stir of life within the womb, a feeling that defies words—there is a physical spark of excitement that echoes straight to your heart. This is the moment you realize your life is no longer your own. You are now carrying the future of another soul within the sanctuary of your heart. Yet, no parent imagines starting their baby's life in the Neonatal Intensive Care Unit (NICU). When it happens, it may feel like your world shatters as you realize the journey ahead is through the NICU rather than the door of your home. But as your old world falls away, a more profound one takes its place. You are finding the path to becoming whole—the ultimate safe harbor for a miracle only you can provide.

The Call to Nursing

My nursing journey did not begin at the bedside; it began on a sunny day in 2001, on the English Literature and Language block of my high school in Jamaica. I was only 13 years old, but I remember the air—thick with humidity and the weight of a life-altering choice—carried a sudden clarity. At that crossroads, I needed to decide on a profession, knowing that choosing prerequisites would ultimately decide my vocational fate. While others were choosing classes, I was choosing a mission.

For a long time, my dream was to become a flight attendant because I wanted to see the world and connect with people. But I realized that I was not just seeking a journey; I was looking for **purpose**. I chose nursing because there was a distinct call on my life for higher service—one that moved me from the cabin of a plane to the bedside of a warrior. Nursing was the vehicle to carry the depth of that offering. In 2006, my university journey began, and on July 10, 2010, I officially held the lamp of responsibility as a Registered General Nurse (RGN). I stepped into this new world with a vow to strive, to serve, and not to yield—the enduring motto of my high school alma mater, *Niti Sevire, Neque Cedere*. This was not just a random promise or a mere sentiment, but what would become the heartbeat of my practice over the next sixteen years of advocacy, service, and resilience.

My clinical foundation was forged over nine years of comprehensive adult and pediatric care, representing a deep culmination of expertise across Medical-Surgical, Orthopedic, Gynecological, and Pediatric units. In 2013, I received certification as a Pediatric and Venipuncture Nurse; that shift launched me into managerial and supervisory roles, but my passion has always been leading from the patient's side.

This near-decade of diverse service sharpened my ability to manage complex systemic pathologies and provided the rigorous groundwork necessary for my transition into the critical-care landscape of the NICU, and I can assuredly say I have no regrets.

Over the years, my clinical eye began to sharpen—a transformation that only occurs through thousands of hours spent in the quiet stillness by a patient's side. It is a specialized intuition that allows a nurse to hear what is not being said and see a change in a baby's status before the monitors even catch the trend. It is the ability to walk into a room and instantly sense the atmospheric shift in your baby's perfusion, the subtle change in a respiratory pattern, or the minute fatigue in a tiny muscle.

This sharpening was forged in the fire of critical adult care and refined in the delicate, high-velocity world of a Pediatric Flight and Ambulance Transport Nurse. It stemmed from a sixteen-year evolution—moving from the checklists of a novice to the seasoned discernment of an expert who can anticipate the storm before the first drop of rain falls.

Why the NICU?

Many have asked why anyone would intentionally choose a world defined by high-stakes silence and the constant tension of the ledge—that thin line between fear and fortitude. The precise moment where you realize that while the machines are loud, your presence is the most powerful force in the room. I chose the NICU because this incredibly vulnerable population is without a voice. They rely solely on the strength of those who have navigated the gap and accepted the mantle of being their primary advocates.

It is in the NICU that we are consistently humbled by the fragility of life yet empowered by the sheer resilience of the human spirit. In this space, we do not just provide medical care; we offer that same humility and empowerment to families walking this journey with us, as your NICU team.

Skill and Soul

While I hold empathy as a sacred pillar of my practice, it is not the only tool in my kit. For the NICU nurse, empathy is tempered by rigorous clinical judgment and high-level technical skill. The heart and the hardware must work in perfect synergy.

Compassion allows me to connect with a terrified parent, but it is clinical judgment that keeps patients safe. If we lead with empathy alone, we risk the weight of overwhelm. And, if we lead with only skill, we provide care that is technically sound but emotionally hollow. To lose empathy makes care mediocre; lacking clinical excellence makes the service dangerous. As NICU nurses, we strive to be as sharp in our assessment as we are soft in our approach.

Perspective from the Heart

After moving to the USA, I spent six years serving as a NICU nurse following a culturally diverse medical-surgical contract in Georgia and Oklahoma. During my time in the NICU, I have witnessed the helplessness, heavy desperation, and grief that mothers and fathers carry as they journey with their babies toward wholeness.

This experience taught me to value every moment: to serve with as much heart as competence, and to lead with grace, empathy, and integrity.

As a parent, I understand the weight of watching helplessly as your baby fights battles that you wish you could fight for them. I can only imagine that moment you learn your baby needs intensive care, how everything shifts, shattering your world. Instead of quiet moments at home, cuddling your baby, you are navigating monitors, medical jargon, and agonizing uncertainty. Fear and exhaustion may accompany this experience, but so do hope and healing.

For The Love Of NICU: Where the Heart Breaks Open and Healing Begins offers invaluable information about the NICU journey. It shares how to gain support and reassures you, as parents, that you are never alone. In these pages, you will find stories from NICU families, and practical strategies for the journey ahead—whether that means bringing your baby home, navigating long-term care, or coping with loss.

Whether your baby is in the NICU for days, weeks, or months, you may feel helpless, scared, or guilty. You might be juggling other children, work, or financial stress. These feelings are completely normal.

But...You are not alone.

While the NICU may not be where you expected to begin parenthood, your love and resilience are already shaping your baby's story.

You are stronger than you think.

CHAPTER 1

The Shock of the Unexpected

In the quiet hum of the NICU, the monitors tell us how your baby's little body is fighting, but only a parent's heart knows how the soul is holding on.

It started with a name. Whether it was Willow, Daniel, Grace, Joshua, Maya, Rhyan, Jalen—before the monitors, before the sterile scent of the NICU, and before the specialized medical terminology, there was simply a life that demanded to be seen.

The journey to the NICU is never a chosen path; it could be an abrupt detour into a world of clinical complexity. Maybe your baby came earlier than expected, was born with a lung or heart condition, had trouble breathing at birth, or needed surgery right away. The entry into the NICU is a moment when the medical "why" suddenly takes center stage.

In an instant, your world is filled with complicated terms, such as respiratory distress or blood infections. These are just words the medical team uses to explain your baby's current status. They are not meant to explain the tiny soul behind *who* your baby is. While the *Pit Crew* of doctors, nurses, therapists, and other support staff focus on the medical labels to provide the best care, remember that these medical labels only define the condition, not your baby. In the NICU, we often speak in the language of data: gestational age, birth weight, and oxygen saturation levels. But behind every set of numbers is a tiny soul that has already rearranged the world of everyone they touch. For parents standing at the bedside, the data doesn't matter nearly as much as the sheer, overwhelming shock of being here at all. The shock of this place may shatter your expectations, but remember: a heart that breaks open is simply making room for a strength it never knew it needed.

Nothing prepares you for this moment.

My professional evolution into caring for the most fragile newborns began over sixteen years ago in Jamaica. At the time, I believed I understood the nature of nursing. I had the clinical training, the sharpened *clinical eye* from pediatric flight transport, and a deep desire to heal. But it wasn't until I stepped onto the pressure-filled NICU stage that I realized I was not just there to treat patients. I was there to witness the exact moment when a family's *expected* life collided with a reality they had not prepared for, and to guide them to a place of safety and healing. Healing does not come from having all the answers. It comes from feeling seen, informed, and supported—moment by moment.

My novice nursing years taught me the most challenging lesson of all: how to maintain clinical excellence while holding space for a family's total *shattering* of expectations. Today, as a Clinical Instructor and Healthcare Simulation Educator, I use clinical scenarios to bridge the gap between theory and practice and teach new nurses to do the same.

Yet...nothing prepares you for this moment.

You may have imagined first cuddles, going-home outfits, a lovingly decorated nursery, and your baby meeting their sibling(s). Maybe you planned a celebration (e.g., christening) within a week or a month of going home. Instead, you are surrounded by beeping monitors, IV pumps, and closed isolettes (incubators). Doctors and nurses use unfamiliar terms *(some of which are provided in Appendix A – The Language of the Pit Crew within this book).* It may feel as though your baby is being cared for in a classroom rather than a nursery because you are told when to hold, feed, or change your baby. You may feel frustrated, overwhelmed, angry, or simply exhausted.

Feel what you must and heal how you can.

The Sensory Landscape of the NICU

When you first walk through the double doors of the NICU, your senses may instantly be pulled into a place that feels completely foreign. Yet, it is here—amidst the beeps and wires—that you will see the quietest, most beautiful miracles happen.

As a Healthcare Simulation Educator, I know that our environment often dictates behavior, and the NICU has its own rhythm, smell, and language. It can create a sensory overload that may leave you feeling untethered. Rest assured, you are not alone. I have identified and shared some of the core sensory experiences of the NICU.

The Sight: Instead of soft blankets and dim lighting, you are met with the sterile glow of fluorescent lights and an intricate web of wires and sensors. I can only imagine the weight of that moment—the heartache of not being able to see your *baby* through the image of the *patient*. In one instance, you are looking at the baby you prepared for—the one you imagined in soft blankets and a beautifully painted nursery. In another, you are looking at the *patient* covered in wires and tape.

It is a sensory wall that may feel impossible to climb, but know that your baby is still there, beneath the plastic of an incubator, the tape, and the wires. When this happens, I would like you to remember this: the machines are only there to watch the body. While the monitor can track a heartbeat, only your voice can soothe; a sensor can measure oxygen, but only your scent can stabilize your baby. The equipment is the hardware of their survival, but you are the heartbeat of their life.

Remember, your love is the only thing the monitors cannot measure. So, when you look past the wires and whisper your baby's name, you are reminding the world—and yourself—that behind every beep, every statistic, and every tube, is a tiny soul that demands to be seen. You are not a spectator—you are the sanctuary for your baby.

The Sound: The rhythmic *whoosh* of ventilators, the sharp, persistent *beep* of an IV or feeding pump, and the hushed, urgent tones of the medical team. This is the "medical jargon" of sound—language that feels cold and foreign when all you crave is the subtle silence of your baby sleeping in their nursery at home. *But listen closer: among the alarms is the steady, quiet thrum of life. Every beep is a sentinel, a tiny guardian telling us your baby is here, they are fighting, and they are not alone.*

The Smell: It is the scent that lingers long after you leave the unit—the sharp, clinical cocktail of rubbing alcohol, hand sanitizer, and industrial-grade detergents. It is a sterile "clean" that lacks the sweet, milky warmth of a home nursery. *Yet, even here, there is a different scent of hope: the faint, earthy smell of your own skin during kangaroo care (skin-to-skin), or the liquid gold of breastmilk being prepared. These are the scents of connection that belong only to you.*

The Touch: You are taught to "hand swaddle" (wrapping your baby securely in a blanket to provide comfort) or "finger hold" (gently grasping your baby's hand for comfort and to enhance the parental bond) through small portholes rather than scooping your baby up to your chest. The plastic of the isolettes (incubators) can feel like a mountain standing between you and your child. *But do not let the equipment deceive you. Your touch is a spiritual connection that no monitor can replicate, and no professional can replace.* When you lay your hand on your baby, you are providing a signature of belonging. Whether it is a mother's heartbeat or a father's steady hand, your baby knows the difference. In a world of sterile surfaces, your touch is the only thing that feels like home.

A Shift in Expectations

The birth of a baby should be a celebration. In the NICU, that celebration is often postponed or muted. You might not get the balloons, streamers, and banners; instead, you get handwashing stations and quiet prayers.

Know that love is still here.

You are not broken, and neither is your baby. You are both in survival mode, and you are doing better than you think. Your strength is not in pretending everything is fine; it is in showing up, loving fiercely, and holding on to hope, even on the most challenging days.

Understanding the Trauma

NICU parents often experience trauma, even when things eventually turn out well. This trauma might stem from the birth itself, the fear of losing your baby, or the constant, agonizing uncertainty. You might smile on the outside while unraveling inside.

Trauma shows up differently for everyone. You might struggle with sleep or having intrusive thoughts. These aren't weaknesses; they are your brain's natural response to extreme stress. You deserve support, not shame. Your *Pit Crew* is here to offer the resources you need to navigate these experiences and refer you to additional support services.

Permission to Feel

In these first few hours and days, I want to give you something the medical monitors cannot—*Permission*. I give you permission to feel the *guilt*—the *"what did I do wrong?"* that haunts the quiet moments. Permission to feel the *Numbness*—that protective wall your brain builds when trauma is too loud. Permission to feel the *Anger*—the rightful sting of a *stolen* beginning.

These feelings are not a sign of weakness; they are a sign of your love. You are grieving the *expected* so that you can eventually embrace the *actual*.

> *"I didn't even get to see his face before they took him away. I kept asking if he was okay, and no one could give me a definite answer. I felt completely powerless."*

A NICU parent

This echoes true for so many NICU parents. Imagine giving birth and not being able to even see or hold your baby. You may immediately imagine the worst or feel instantly thrust into a traumatic journey. You are not alone. Give yourself permission to feel everything.

First Steps Forward

In these early days, give yourself permission to mourn the beginning you expected.

Ask questions, no matter how repetitive they feel.

Take breaths and take breaks. Your baby needs you to be healthy.

Let others help you. You were never meant to go this journey alone.

Feel whatever you're feeling. It is okay if you don't "feel" like a parent right away. It is okay if you feel scared. It is *all* okay.

Showing up is enough right now—and you are showing up. In time, this will become part of your story, but it is not the whole story. For now, just breathe. Be gentle with yourself. There is no right way to cope—there is only **your** way.

This journey may be unexpected or new to you—many have walked similar paths before you and stand as a testament. I would like you to remember that you are not alone, even if it feels that way.

NOTES

I invite you to take a moment to write your heart steady, anchor your mind, and claim the peace that belongs to you in this very moment.

CHAPTER 2

Life Inside the NICU

The NICU is a place suspended between fear and hope, science and miracles.

I understand the weight of watching a hospital become your *"second home."* For many parents, it becomes an unfamiliar world you never wanted to enter, but cannot imagine leaving until your baby is well enough to go home safely in your arms. It is a world where the walls are made of glass, the lullabies are replaced by rhythmic beeps, and you are learning to be a parent while simultaneously learning a new medical language. To navigate this landscape, you need more than just hope; you need *clarity*.

What is the NICU?

To the outside world, the Neonatal Intensive Care Unit (NICU) is a hospital department. But to those of us inside, it is a specialized environment designed to finish the work the womb started; I invite you to think of it as a protective bridge for your baby, a place of solace and safety.

The External Womb

For many babies, the NICU acts as a high-tech extension of the pregnancy, like an external womb.

The Isolette (Incubator): provides the warmth and humidity of the womb.

Monitors and machines: track your baby's heart rate, breathing, oxygen levels, and blood pressure. They are like an extension of the womb that once helped to sustain life and provide protection. Alarms sound frequently, but they do not always signal danger—often they just mean something needs adjustment.

Tubes and Wires:

- *IV lines* provide fluids to hydrate your baby or give additional nutrition needed for growth and development.
- *Oxygen cannulas or ventilators* provide support for your baby's growing lungs. Each one helps your baby grow stronger.
- *The Feeding Tubes* provide the nutrition previously delivered by the umbilical cord.
- *Respiratory Support* does the work that developing lungs are not yet strong enough to do alone.

The Observation Deck

The *Intensive* in NICU means your baby is being watched with incredible precision. This constant stream of data is a shield of **safety**. We use technology to detect the *whispers* of change before they become a shout, allowing us to adjust the "blueprints" of your baby's care in real time.

Your Elite Pit Crew

In the NICU, your baby's care team does not just have a doctor; they have a multidisciplinary team of specialists. Understanding the different roles helps you know who to turn to with your questions as you build your baby's bridge home.

The Neonatologist: This is the lead doctor who oversees your baby's entire medical plan and long-term goals.

The Neonatal Nurse Practitioner (NNP): They are the advanced practice nurses who are the *boots on the ground*, managing daily shifts in care and clinical decisions for your baby.

The Bedside Nurse: They are your primary partner. They know the personality of your baby and are your first line of communication.

The Respiratory Therapist (RT): They are experts in everything involving breathing and lung health, and the machines that support them.

The Occupational/Physical Therapist (OT/PT): They focus on your baby's development, positioning, and first feedings.

Speech-Language Pathologist (SLP): You might wonder why a speech therapist is seeing a baby who cannot talk yet. In the NICU, these specialists are experts in feeding and swallowing. They understand the intricate coordination of sucking, swallowing, and breathing. They help determine when your baby is ready for the breast or a bottle, ensuring every drop is a safe and successful step toward home.

The Lactation Consultant: They are the professional champions of the breast-feeding and pumping journey. They provide the "know-how" and emotional support to help provide your baby with the liquid gold they need.

The Social Worker: Think of them as your family navigator. They are not here because something is wrong; they are here to help you manage the logistical and emotional weight of your NICU stay. They assist you with everything from insurance and discharge planning to connecting with mental health resources and support groups to help you.

The Dietitian/Nutritionist: This is your baby's fuel specialist. They work behind the scenes to help calculate the exact balance of proteins, fats, and vitamins your baby needs to grow.

I encourage you to rest in the precision of their work; they are meticulously crafting the physical strength your baby will one day use to run into your arms.

The Daily Routine

The NICU runs on tight schedules—feeding times, medication rounds, temperature checks, and monitoring are carefully choreographed. You will quickly learn terms like oxygen saturation, jaundice (yellowing of the skin), and bradycardia/brady events (a decrease in heart rate). *Remember that you are the only part of this routine that your baby truly knows by heart.*

The Emotional Roller Coaster

Being in the NICU is like riding a roller coaster you never bought a ticket for. There was no slow climb to prepare you; instead, you are dropped into the first dip before you can even catch your breath.

There are *Loop-the-Loop* days where a new alarm sounds, and you feel that stomach-flipping drop. It is the feeling of being in a freefall where you are bracing for impact, waiting for the *Pit Crew* to stabilize the care, so you can find your level ground again. It is here that your role solidifies from spectator to a partner in your baby's care.

Then there are the ebbs—those long quiet stretches when it seems nothing is moving. It may feel like you are adrift in a calm but foggy sea. The adrenaline of the initial crisis has worn off, but the relief of going home is still out of sight. These moments may feel taxing in a different way; they require a marathon mindset to keep rowing when you cannot seem to see the shore. On days like these, give yourself permission to recharge your battery: go on short walks, close your eyes, and rest. This is a requirement because every warrior needs to be ready for the next climb.

And then there are the peaks. These are days where your baby thrives, their breathing tube is removed, you get to hold them skin-to-skin for the first time, or they reach their goal weight. These are summits where the air feels clear again. It is the surge of hope that reminds you why you are fighting.

During the downturns, it is tempting to retreat—sit back, stay on your phone, or talk loudly to distract yourself. But the ride is steadier when you are in the driver's seat by remaining present and aware of changes in your baby's condition and know it is always okay to voice your concerns and seek clarification from your *Pit Crew*.

The Vital Role of Parents

Throughout your time in the NICU, you may feel like a visitor—please know that you are not visitors here; you are biological necessities. While the team manages clinical care, both parents provide a biological connection that no machine can replicate. You are the heart of the team, and we welcome your presence and your voice.

Your presence and involvement are powerful.

The Power of Your Combined Presence

Your baby knows the rhythm of your heart. Research shows that infants respond uniquely to the different frequencies of a mother's and a father's voice.[1] It promotes the development of language pathways in your baby's brain and enhances communication skills and cognitive development.

The Sound of Home: As parents, you are encouraged to talk, sing, or read to your baby. Your voices are familiar melodies that lower their stress hormones and stabilize their heart rates. Talk and sing to your baby—they recognize your voice. Reading quietly or singing comforts them and supports their development.

The Gift of Silence: High-pitched or loud talking can be overstimulating to your baby. Both parents should practice using a *hushed, nursery voice* to protect the baby's sanctuary of sleep. Quality sleep is necessary for physical growth, maintenance of a healthy weight, and brain development while helping to reduce the risk of illness.

The *No-Phone* Sanctuary: When you are at the bedside, it is advised to keep your phone silent and tucked away. The blue light and constant *pings* are overstimulating for a developing nervous system. Use this time to be fully present; your baby feels that focused energy.

---

1. Scientific studies have shown that your baby is not just hearing noise; they are tuned into the specific rhythm and pitch of your voice. Research confirms that even tiny infants can distinguish their parent's unique frequencies from the background of the hospital. While the mother's voice offers a familiar melody from the womb, the father's distinct tones provide a biological signal that tells your baby they are not alone (DeCasper & Fifer, 1980). Full reference:DeCasper, A. J., & Fifer, W. P. (1980). Of human bonding: Newborns prefer their mother's voices. Science, 208 (4448), 1174 -1176. https://doi.org/10.1126/science.7375928.

Bonding With Your Baby Through Touch

If your baby is too fragile to be held. Your touch can regulate their heartbeat, temperature, and breathing. Know that it is safe to ask questions because none of your questions or concerns are too small or insignificant; this allows you to take joint ownership of the blueprint for your baby's care.

Participating as Collaborative Architects

Both parents should feel empowered to participate in "Cares" (the scheduled times we change, assess, and feed your baby). As your baby stabilizes, you will be encouraged to help with diaper changes, feeding, bathing, and temperature checks. These moments build your confidence and your bond.

Small Victories

Milestones look different in the NICU. Every small victory deserves recognition and celebration. Even when your baby gains an ounce, it is cause for celebration. Progress might look like:

- Gaining weight consistently for 3 days or more.
- Tolerating consistent feedings.
- Coming off oxygen support for good.
- Regulating body temperature without support.
- The first bath, first clothes, or first time being held.

Every step matters. These little warriors fight battles measured in grams and breaths. Celebrate them and you.

Preparing to Go Home

Discharge from the NICU is not just a release—it is a graduation. You may feel joy mixed with fear. Joy because your baby finally gets to go home, and fear because there are no more machines to alert you. Know that nurses are close by or a button-press away. Before your baby comes home with you, the team prepares you by ensuring:

- Your baby can breathe and feed independently.
- Your baby is gaining weight steadily.
- You are confident in caring for your baby.

Steps are in place to support your growth in confidence, including CPR training and infant safety training, which are available to you. Plus, any equipment and usage guides will be supplied to you, including monitors, medications, and feeding supplies. Guidance is also offered for follow-up appointments. You will leave stronger, more vigilant, more confident, and attuned. And your baby leaves with an unshakable will.

A Note for Your Hearts as Parents

On the days when the emotional roller coaster feels too fast, remember, as parents, whether you are a couple or a solo parent, you are the only people who are not 'at work.' You are the only people who are *home* to your baby. When you engage—sing, touch, and hold your baby and ask questions—you are not just guests. You are the steady ground your baby is reaching for. Even if you feel shaky, or are doing this journey without a partner, you are the anchor for your baby. Trust the bond that exists beneath the surface.

We are right here with you.

NOTES

I invite you to take a moment to write your heart steady, anchor your mind, and claim the peace that belongs to you in this very moment.

CHAPTER 3

Coping with Emotional Overwhelm

The NICU is a place of forced contradictions. You may feel the weight of a heavy heart and the lift of a tiny victory in the very same breath.

Within the enclosed walls of the NICU exists a strange, fervent middle space, a place of incredible contradiction where your heart is asked to stretch in opposite directions simultaneously. We call it the *NICU Paradox*. This is one of the most confusing emotional landscapes a parent will ever navigate. It is the jarring reality of holding two conflicting truths at the same time—feeling both grateful for the technology saving your baby and heartbroken that they need it in the first place.

I understand how these words might feel as you read them. It may feel unsettling to realize at once. But I would like you to take a deep breath and hear the truth behind that contradiction:

You are safe to feel all the emotions that are often enveloped in the NICU experience.

Finding clarity in this divide is the first step toward managing the overwhelm that comes with it.

Gratitude and Grief: You may be deeply thankful for the Pit Crew and the life-saving machines, yet you feel grief for the normal and uneventful birth you expected and the nursery you hoped for.

Intimacy and Distance: You have never been more connected to your child's every breath, yet you may feel miles away because you must ask permission to touch them through a porthole.

Strength and Fragility: You are witnessing the absolute power of your little warrior, even as they look so incredibly small against the backdrop of the machines. But remember, you are your little Warrior's Warrior. You are the strength behind their struggle and the voice for their fight.

Saying your heart feels *full* is not defining a state of brokenness but rather an acknowledgement of how much love you carry. *Tiny victories* point to the immense strength you and your baby already possess. This paradox is not a trap; it is a testament to your capacity as a parent. You are your little warrior's warrior. You are being held in this moment by a team that understands this tension. You do not have to choose between being *strong* and feeling *sad*. You are allowed to feel both, and in that honesty, you are protected.

Defining the NICU Paradox: Joy and Grief

We are taught that *joy* and *grief* live in different houses. We may be tempted to think we have to finish grieving before we can start being joyful. The opposite is true; both can coexist in our hearts. In the NICU, these two are roommates; they share the same space, the same breath, and the same heart. Understanding them allows you to master this journey with more clarity, courage, and hope.

What is Joy in the NICU?

In the NICU, joy does not usually look like a big, loud celebration. It is a moment of soft, quiet elation. It is found in the stillness of a stable hour and a steady rhythm of a tiny life.

The Relief of a Stable Hour: It is at that moment the doctor walks away and says, *"Everything looks good for now."* It is the deep exhale you did not know you were holding.

The Miracle of the Smallest Things: It is a single milliliter (ml) of milk digested. It is a tiny finger curling around yours. It is the nurse leaning in to whisper that your baby ate 2 milliliters from a bottle for the first time—and did great—or informing you how well your baby did after coming off oxygen. These are the milestones that build the bridge to home.

The Home in Your Heart: It is the realization that, despite the wires and the plastic walls of an isolette (incubator), this is your baby. It is the sudden fierce surge of love that tells you that no matter how small they are, they win marathons and move mountains; they are a giant in your world.

What is Grief in the NICU?

Grief here is often misunderstood because your baby is right in front of you. It is not only about the passing of a loved one. It is about lost expectations, dreams deferred, and plans shattered. You are allowed to grieve the birth story you wanted, the newborn photos you did not get, or the easy start you imagined. Grief is not who you *are*; it is a response to the shattering of the story you expected.

The Longing for the *Normal*: It is the sting you feel when someone shares a "coming home" post on social media or the ache of an empty nursery at home while you sit in a hospital chair.

The Weight of *What-Ifs*: It is the exhaustion of playing out a hundred different scenarios in your head. It is the sadness of not being the first one to hold, bathe, or dress your baby.

The Fatigue of the Unknown: It is the *fog* that settles over you when the medical jargon gets too loud. It is the feeling of being a *visitor* in your own baby's life.

We often think of these emotions as opposites, and you might feel like you are betraying your baby by feeling sad or betraying your reality by feeling joyful. Realizing that the deepest ache and the highest joy can occupy the same room is the solemnity of the NICU Paradox. You do not have to wait for the pain and sadness to disappear before you let love in.

You can grieve and love at the same time. You can learn to embrace the NICU Paradox now that you understand it.

Your Grounding Toolkit for Moments of Chaos

When you are in the NICU, your *"fight-or-flight response"* is active. Having a calming toolkit to call upon will support your nervous system during this chaotic time. These techniques are not just "distractions"—they are biological resets. These are evidence-based, reliable methods used by medical professionals to send signals to your brain that you are safe. Try these techniques and see which work best for you. Use them when you need that extra support to ground yourself.

Tapping into the "Brake Pedal"

The Science of the Autonomic Nervous System: Your body has an *Automatic Pilot* called the autonomic nervous system. It controls things like your heartbeat and digestion, and it has two main settings:

The Gas Pedal (Sympathetic): This is your "Fight-or-Flight" response which revs you up and gets you moving or remaining still.

The Brake Pedal (Parasympathetic): This is "Rest and Digest," which calms you down.

In the NICU, your body can get stuck with its foot slammed on the gas pedal. These techniques act as the Brake Pedal, helping your body return to a state where it can actually rest and feel grounded.

Clearing the Stress Messenger (Cortisol)

The Science of Cortisol: Cortisol is your body's built-in alarm hormone. It helps you handle an emergency in short bursts. But when you stay in the NICU for days or weeks, your body produces too much for too long, leaving you feeling *wired, tired,* or *shaky*. When you use these tools to lower your cortisol, you are clearing the *stress chemicals* out of your blood so you can feel more like yourself again.

Positive Affirmations for the Soul

Healing begins when you choose to stop claiming the achy pain as your identity. You are not the weight of your anxiety, sadness, guilt, resentment, or helplessness; you are a parent experiencing a difficult moment. When the shadows feel heavy, use these positive affirmations to anchor your mind in the truth of your strength:

I feel the depth of my love for my baby in every breath I take.
I am the perfect parent for my baby, and my presence is their greatest comfort.
I trust my baby's resilience and the expertise of our care team.
I am capable of navigating this journey with grace and steady hope.
My bond with my baby is unbreakable, eternal, and growing stronger every day.

I now invite you to close your eyes and imagine your heart is like a wide, open meadow or a slow, steady stream. You may feel the rain of a challenging day, but the rain does not change the fact that the sun is still there, waiting, anchored, and ready to break through. You do not need the rain to stop for the sun to be real. Both can exist at once. When you allow yourself to say, ***"I feel the weight of this experience, and I am head-over-heels in love with this amazing little human of mine,"*** you are no longer divided. *You are whole.*

Your Survival Trio: The Essential Grounding Tools

While there are many techniques used in clinical settings to manage stress, focusing on these three specific tools will prove most beneficial for your journey. They have been selected because they can be done right at the bedside, and address both your mind and body.

Since you are already learning a new medical language and navigating a complex environment, you do not need a long list of "to-dos." You need a reliable kit that works every single time.

Think of these as your *emotional monitors*. Just as we watch your baby's vital signs (heart rate, temperature, oxygen level, blood pressure), these tools help you monitor and steady your own.

1. 5-4-3-2-1 Grounding Method

The Science of Sensory-Motor Grounding: Think of your brain like a computer with too many tabs open. When you feel anxious, your mind is stuck in internal tabs—the scary "what-if" thoughts. Sensory-motor grounding is like hitting the Refresh button. By forcing your brain to notice things you see, feel, hear, smell, and taste, you will pull your energy away from those scary thoughts and plug back into the physical world. Your brain is then reminded to pause and focus on the here and now—inviting you to stop looking at the what-ifs and start looking at the what-is.

The Purpose

The technique uses sensorimotor grounding to interrupt a panic spiral by engaging the logical part of your brain.

How to Use

Sit or stand still and bring your awareness into your immediate surroundings.

Acknowledge 5 things you see.

Acknowledge 4 things you can touch.

Acknowledge 3 things you hear.

Acknowledge 2 things you can smell.

Acknowledge 1 thing you can taste.

Take a deep breath and embrace the stillness of the moment.

2. Box Breathing (Square Breathing)

The Science of the *Logical Brain*: In a crisis, your *Survival Brain* runs the show. This is the part of your brain that stays alert for alarms. It cannot think clearly while it tries to protect you. Your *Logical Brain* is the part that processes information and makes decisions. When you do *Box Breathing*, you physically force the *Survival Brain* to step down so the *Logical Brain* can take the wheel again.

The Purpose

This regulates the autonomic nervous system, lowering your heart rate and reducing cortisol.

How to Use

Visualize a square.

Inhale for 4 seconds.

Hold for 4 seconds.

Exhale for 4 seconds.

Hold the empty breath for 4 seconds.

Repeat 4 times.

3. Journaling

For a NICU parent, your mind may feel like a crowded room where everyone is shouting at once. Journaling is the act of taking those voices and giving them a seat. It is a clinical tool for emotional regulation that moves your experiences from a *tangled knot* in your chest to a *story* on the page.

As a trusted friend sitting in that chair next to you, let me share a secret: you do not need to be a writer to do this. There is no right way to journal, and you definitely do not need structure or form. You are offloading what is on your heart. Whether it is a single word, a messy list, or just a scribble of how you are feeling right now, let the paper hold the weight so you do not have to. Allow the ink to flow—because in this space, the only *perfect* words are the ones that come from the depth of your soul—the quiet fears, the hope, the grief, the joy, the anger, the resilience, the now.

Free Flowing Journal

When you write down the fears, joys, and the 2 ml victories, you are engaging in *Expressive Writing.*

The Purpose

Research shows that labeling your emotion reduces the activity in the *Survival Brain* (the Amygdala) and increases activity in the *Logical Brain.*[1] It lowers your

1. Lieberman, M. D., et al. (2007). Putting feelings into words: Affect labeling disrupts amygdala activity in response to affective stimuli. Psychological Science, 18(5), 421-428.

heart rate and helps your immune system stay strong during the stress of the hospital stay. It is a way of "offloading" the trauma so your mind doesn't have to carry it all.

How To Use

You do not need a fancy notebook—the back of a parking receipt or a notes application on your phone works just as well. The goal is to release the weight in your chest, the quiet fears that keep you up at night, and the heavy feelings, so you can make room for the soft elation.

The Right Now Prompts: The following prompts can be used when you are feeling overwhelmed by answering the following:

Right now, the loudest thought in my head is...

I feel the most steady when...

If I didn't have to be brave for anyone else right now, I would say that I feel...

One thing I wish the medical team knew about me today is ...

I am giving myself permission to feel...

If I could change one thing about today's routine, it would be...

The first thing we are going to do together when we finally get home is...

The Baby's Breath Prompts

The following prompts can be used when you are in need of connecting with your baby:

One tiny thing my baby did today that showed their strength was...

When I looked at my baby today, I noticed...

I feel my bond with my baby growing when we...

The most beautiful part of my baby's face today was...

When I look at my baby, the one detail I want to remember forever is...

The first time I touched my baby's skin or hand, I felt...

The first promise I made to my baby in my heart was...

The Victory Log

The following prompts can be used when you have something to celebrate your baby being closer to the bridge to home:

Today's "2 ml victory" was...

One question I asked today that made me feel like a partner in my baby's care was...

One thing I did today to take care of myself as "the parent" was...

Today I stopped worrying about the monitors for a moment and instead focused on...

One thing my baby did today that proved they are a fighter is...

A moment today where I felt my own Warrior's Warrior strength kick in was when I...

A Healing Perspective

You might feel like you do not have the energy to write. That is okay. Some days, a journal entry might just be one word: *Exhausted*. Other days it might be a letter to your baby that they will read ten years from now.

There is no wrong or right way to do this. **You are the author of this journey**. By writing it down, you are claiming your story. You are moving from feeling like a visitor in the unit to the *Chronicler* of your family's resilience.

A Note from the Bedside: The Connection Beneath the Surface

If I could pull up a chair next to yours for just a moment, take a deep breath with you, and share what I've learned over the past sixteen years, this is what I would say ...

You are supported. You have an entire team that is not just watching over and taking care of your baby—we are watching over you. We are the *Collaborative Architects* of this journey. It is okay to lean on us; okay to let us carry the medical burden so you can simply be a parent.

You are safe. The NICU is a sanctuary not just for your baby—it is also a sanctuary for you, too. Every alarm is a promise that we are paying attention. Every sterile drape is a shield we have placed around your family. You are allowed to let down your guard. You are allowed to breathe. We are here for you.

There is a profound connection that exists entirely outside of what we can physically see on a monitor. Your baby's primary environment is not the hospital—it is you. When you sit at the bedside, even if you are not speaking to or touching your baby, your presence matters. This is the intuitive bond that tells your baby they belong to someone, they belong to you, they are loved, and they are not alone.

You are resilient, you are loved, and you are doing better than you think. Give yourself grace. Trust the bond that exists beneath the surface. We are right here with you always.

NOTES

I invite you to take a moment to write your heart steady, anchor your mind, and claim the peace that belongs to you in this very moment.

Chapter 4

Finding Your Role as a Parent

You are a new parent to your little warrior, yet you may feel like a guest in a sterile room.

The nurses handle the clinical care, the doctors make the medical decisions, and you might feel as though the unit runs just as well whether you are there or not. I invite you to see a deeper truth: *while we provide medical intervention, you provide the biological home*. You are not a visitor. You are the parent, and your role is the only one in this room that is irreplaceable.

The Shift from Spectator to Primary Anchor

For the first few days, it is natural to stand back. You are processing a lot, and the hum of the monitors can feel like a wall between you and your baby. The most profound shift in your journey happens when you realize that the medical team is supporting your baby. We are the technicians, but you are the *Chief Architect.*

Your role is not just to watch; it is to provide the environment that supports your baby's brain development. You are the bridge between a high-tech hospital and the life that awaits you at home.

Your Superpowers Defined

In the medical world, we use big words like **Neuro-protective Care**, but all that means is **protecting the brain.** Every time you choose to be quiet at the bedside, every time you touch your baby, you are shielding their developing brain from the stress of the hospital environment.

You are the filter that lets the good in and keeps the scary things out because your superpowers are remarkable; the depth of your being encompasses the biological regulator, human thermostat, and metronome. You are a powerful source for your baby.

The Biological Regulator

When you practice kangaroo care (skin-to-skin), your body is doing the thinking for your baby's body. You become their biological regulator, helping them to be at their best temperature.

The *Human Thermostat*

There is a miracle of nature called *Thermal Synchronization.* When you hold your baby against your bare skin, your chest acts like a smart thermostat. If your baby is too cold, your body heat rises to warm them up. If they are running a fever, your skin cools down to help them. This is your body's way of syncing your temperature to theirs to keep them safe.

The *Metronome Effect*

Your steady heartbeat and your rhythmic breathing act like a metronome for a musician. Your baby listens to your body and follows your lead. It helps their own heart and lungs find a steady, calm rhythm.

The human body is fascinating, and as you witness your tiny baby marvel at you, remember you are also a marvel to them.

The Womb Hug

When a baby is very small or fragile, they can feel "lost" in the open space of an isolette (incubator). The womb hug makes them feel safe. It is also called the containment hold.

The Purpose

The Womb Hug recreates the snug, secure feeling of the womb, providing a sense of containment.

The Technique

Think of it as a "still hug." Place your warm, still hands on your baby's head and feet at the same time. Avoid stroking or patting, which can feel like a "tickle" or an irritation to their sensitive skin. A firm, still, loving hold is the most restorative gift you can give to your baby.

The Sound of Safety

Your baby's hearing is one of their most developed senses. In a room filled with mechanical beeps and metallic clicks, your voice is a tether to the familiar.

The Sensory Anchor: Talking, reading, or singing isn't just about entertainment. It is about providing an **anchor**. It tells the baby's nervous system, *"I know this sound. I am safe."* It pulls them out of the medical noise and back into the family.

The Guardian of Rest: Choosing to put the phone away and speaking in hushed tones is a medical choice—rather than reacting to noise, it allows their brain to focus on growth, rest, and recovery.

Advocacy and Intuition

As a nurse, I have seen it countless times. A parent leans over the isolette (incubator), looks at their baby, and says, *"He just seems a little 'off' today."* To an outsider, the monitors might look stable and the charts might look unchanged. But to me, that sentence is a vital clinical signal. *Listen to that voice.* You are the only person in the hospital who is tuned into the frequency of your baby's soul. While you are becoming an expert on your baby's needs, be confident in the fact that your *Pit Crew* are willing to listen to your concerns.

Context Meets Clinical Data

The monitors give us *data* (the numbers), but you give us *context* (the story). While the monitors and the medical team provide **clinical data**, you provide the **essential context**. You are not just noticing things; you are collecting data a machine could never track.

The neonatologists, nurses, and specialists are the experts in the medical field, *how?* They are highly trained eyes and ears that provide continuous, high-level care 24 hours a day. However, your role is to become the expert in your baby's, *who*?

Personality Behind the Pathology

Even in the middle of a crisis, your baby's personality is already demanding to be seen. As you watch them, you begin to recognize who they are becoming.

The Fighter: the baby who pushes back against the wires and keeps the team on their toes.

The Old Soul: The baby who seems to watch the room with a quiet, steady patience.

The Sensitive Spirit: The baby who knows the exact moment your hand touches the glass and settles instantly.

The Circle of Advocacy

Over time, you will learn the tiny, subtle cues – the specific way they hold their hands or a unique eyebrow furrow—that belong only to them.

It is important to share your observations with the team. When you do this, you are not being "difficult." You are adding a vital, personal piece to the medical puzzle.

By partnering with us in this way, we are combining your unique perspective with the team's professional expertise, creating the most complete and safe plan for your baby's journey. A proven partnership that works.

The Final Truth About Helplessness

You might feel helpless because you cannot change the circumstances, but you are never powerless, so do not apologize for your intuition.

You may not be able to fix the lungs or cure the infection—that is the medical team's job. But you can provide love, the scent, or the specific voice that tells your baby they belong and they are loved.

Building Confidence for the Journey Home

You might leave the NICU feeling like you are still learning, and that is okay. Whether your baby was born before 24 weeks (about 5 and a half months) or was a full-term baby who needed unexpected support, the transition to home is a major milestone.

No parent feels 100% ready—even those who have never stepped foot in a NICU.

But look at what you have already mastered.

You have learned to read monitors, handle fragile skin, and navigate a medical landscape most people have never seen.

When it is your baby's time to go home, you will realize you are more ready than you feel, and that matters more than you know.

NOTES

I invite you to take a moment to write your heart steady, anchor your mind, and claim the peace that belongs to you in this very moment.

CHAPTER 5

The NICU Rollercoaster

Progress is not a ladder we climb toward the exit. It is a roller coaster—filled with quiet climbs, sudden drops, and unexpected turns.

The NICU is a journey that rarely follows a straight line, so if you are expecting it to be a predictable climb, it is important to understand that this journey follows a different map. It is a non-linear path. The NICU is not a highway; it is a rugged terrain of peaks and valleys. Whether your journey takes days or months, every twist is a chance to show up for your baby in ways you never knew you could. While this path may challenge your spirit, acknowledging the ups and downs as a natural part of the process is how to begin to find your footing. And remember, the ride does not define your worth as a parent.

We often celebrate the *mountaintop moments*—the first time your baby breathes without the ventilator or the first gain in weight. These milestones are the light that guides the way. But I encourage you to also honor the moments in the valley.

The valleys—*those days of one step forward, two steps back*—are not signs of failure. They are the quiet spaces where your baby is gathering strength. When the path dips, you are not losing ground; you are simply navigating the reality of healing. By making peace with the unpredictable rhythm of the unit, you move from a place of waiting *for it to be over* to a place of unshakable presence.

A valley is just the space between two peaks. Your baby is still moving forward, and even in the low points, you are the steady anchor that keeps them from drifting. Honor the struggle as much as the success, because your *warrior* is forged in the climb.

To truly understand this concept, look at the stories written in these rooms every day—stories that invite us to move beyond our own fear and into a space of empathy and deep gratitude. The story is not written in ink; it is written in the rise and fall of a chest, the grasp of a tiny hand, and the quiet resilience of parents who refuse to leave the side of their miracle. When we look at these stories, we see that the path is not just about medical milestones—it is about the transformation of the soul.

Architect Spotlight: The Cost of the Foundation

"We entered the NICU with twins, but we only went home with one. Losing one twin while the other was still fighting for his life was a grief I can't put into words. It felt like my heart was being pulled in two different directions every single day.

When our surviving son developed complications, and his journey grew longer, the pressure from the outside world—even from my own family—became heavy. They didn't understand why I couldn't just leave him with the nurses or why I was so 'difficult' about his care. I had to make an agonizing choice to pull away from people who couldn't support my role as his advocate. I lost relationships because I chose to be the parent he needed.

I spent those months in the NICU being his anchor and shield. Even when I felt exhausted, I provided skin-to-skin and comforted him with my voice while navigating his new need for home oxygen. It was a long, steep climb, but I stayed the course. Today, watching him thrive at home, I know that every difficult decision and every lost connection was worth the life he is living now. I wasn't just a grieving parent for the son I lost—I was home for the son who stayed."

A NICU Parent

If you are reading this as a parent with a similar story, there is hope and healing in this space. While one of your babies may not be here in presence, their legacy and fight lives on in your heart. You may still be navigating the climb, receiving comfort in knowing that you are your Warrior's Warrior.

Why We Call It a Graduation

In these rooms, *graduation* is not just a cute term for going home. It is a title earned through fire. It marks the moment your baby has mastered the *curriculum* of survival—breathing, feeding, and growing—and the moment *you* have mastered the *curriculum* of advocacy. You are moving from a world of monitors and permissions into the freedom of your own front door.

While graduation is a victory, we honor the fact that for many, it feels bittersweet. It is a complex mix of relief and the weight of leaving the cocoon of the medical team. You may be walking away with your baby, as well as the memory of the struggle you have just gone through. Remember that whether the journey was ten days or ten months, graduation is the celebration of a life that demanded to be seen. It is the moment the tiny soul is no longer a patient, but a son or daughter, finally coming home to a new life forged from a paradox.

The Grace of the Short Surge

Sometimes, the roller coaster is a brief, intense loop. There are parents who arrive at the NICU with their baby at 40 weeks, their hearts set on a standard celebration, only to find themselves in the unit because of a sudden respiratory complication.

For seven days, they lived in a blur of shock. They sat in sterile silence, watching their baby's chest move too fast or too hard, feeling the jarring disconnect between the nursery they prepared and the hospital room they were given.

But then, the breathing eased into normalcy. The monitors went quiet, and they finally walked out the doors with a healthy baby. Their healing comes in the realization that **health is not a guarantee; it is a gift.** Their NICU journey was short in days but long in perspective. It taught them that every breath their baby takes is a miracle they will never take for granted again. When you see a "quick" graduation, let it be a reminder that recovery is a powerful, sacred thing.

The Steady Miracle of a Long Climb

Across the hall, you might see the parents of the 29-weeker who has lived within these walls for 73 days. For them, the roller coaster has been a slow, grueling incline, where progress is measured not in miles, but in millimeters.

They have watched their baby fight for every breath and struggle for every ounce of growth. In this space, healing does not come in a sudden burst; it reveals itself in *the miracle of the small experiences.* These parents have learned to find more profound joy in a tiny weight gain than most parents find in a first birthday party.

Their journey is a masterclass of patience. They serve as a quiet, powerful reminder that the "long road" is often where the deepest, most resilient strength resides.

The Beauty of a Different Destination

There is the family whose roller coaster leads to a home that looks nothing like the one they planned. Their baby arrived at full term, but an unexpected complication at the very end changed their lives "forever." They leave with a journey that continues with significant developmental challenges and a life that moves to a different beat.

Healing for these parents doesn't come from "fixing" a deficit: it comes from *redefining the miracle.* They learn to fall in love with the baby they have, not the one they expected. They find closure by realizing that a smile is a victory, no matter when it happens.

They are the pioneers of a path that requires a deeper, more resilient kind of love. They remind us that thriving does not have a single definition, and that your baby's worth should never be measured by a checklist of milestones.

A Lifetime in Days

In the quietest corner of the unit, we find the journey that ends sooner than we ever imagined. There are parents who enter these doors carrying the weight of losing multiple pregnancies, then finally meeting their son or daughter born at just 22 weeks only to say goodbye to another brave warrior.

Their arrival is a fragile miracle, a tiny life that exists in the delicate space between hope and heartbreak. For these parents, the roller coaster is not a long journey of months, but a poignant, concentrated lifetime of healing from the void their child has left and a loving memory of a child whose warm hold they never clung to.

Their parenting is redefined in those quiet hours. It is not found in the typical milestones of first steps or words, but is a deeper form of love. Because they cannot provide the physical comforts of home in one hold, their devotion becomes an act of pure presence. It is found in the stillness of their hands resting against the thick plastic of the isolette (incubator), and listening to the low hum of their familiar voices—a sound that carries the weight of endless promises in those few days.

When they eventually leave the hospital, their car seat is empty. But as they walk to the parking lot, they hold a small box of memoirs—a tiny hat, a footprint—like it is made of gold. Their story is the hardest turn on the roller coaster, yet it offers the deepest closure for the rest of us.

They were not just grieving the child they lost; they were home for the one who stayed for a moment. They remind us that if they can find peace in those days, we can find the strength to get through today.

When I speak of *"we"*, I am not just referring to the doctors and nurses at the bedside, nor am I only speaking to the parents holding vigil. I am speaking to the unified front that forms around every isolette (incubator)—the *Partnership* of the *Protection*.

"We" is the bridge between the medical chart and the cradle.

To the Parent: "We" is your permission to take your seat at the table. It is the realization that while you may not have a medical degree, you hold the doctorate in your baby's soul.

To the Healthcare Professional: "We" is a reminder that clinical excellence is incomplete without the parent's presence. It is an invitation to see the mother and father not as visitors to be managed, but as the most vital members of the care team.

When we speak, we speak for those who cannot yet speak for themselves. We are the *warrior's warrior*—a collective of experts and advocates, scientists and soul-keepers, all focused on a single, sacred mission: bringing your tiny soul safely home.

Survival Skills for the Ride

While you cannot control the tracks of the roller coaster, you can control how you sit in the seat. Here is your guide to navigating the most difficult drops:

Creating a Digital Sanctuary

Your phone is a wonderful window to the world, but in the NICU, it can also be a source of noise when you need quiet. Use it to capture the small, sacred moments—the way the light hits the isolette (incubator), the curve of a tiny ear, or the first time those eyes flutter open. But if you find yourself scrolling through the lives of others and feeling a weight in your chest, give yourself permission to look away. Your journey is yours alone, and it is beautiful in its own timing. Use your phone to document this miracle, and do not be afraid to set it down when you just want to be present in the stillness.

The Two Steps Forward Invitation

Unexpected complications are not failures; they are the nature of the track. This journey may include an emergency surgery, a sudden need to go back on oxygen support, a transfer to a different facility, or having to stop eating to start IV fluids. These moments can feel like the ground is shifting beneath you, but I invite you to see them differently.

If your baby needs a little extra support today after a great day yesterday, try not to lose heart. It is not a setback; it is a *pause*. Just as a climber stops to catch their breath before the steepest part of the mountain, your baby is simply gathering strength for the next climb. These *stops* are not a sign that you are going backward; they are the moments where your baby's body is recalibrating and preparing for the next victory. *Trust the pause.*

When Others Go Home

There will be days when you see another family packing their bags and dressing their baby in their "going home" outfit. It is okay if your heart feels heavy even as you smile with them. When you see a baby graduate, try to see it as proof that the ride eventually ends. Their joy is a promise that your day is coming too.

The End of the Track

Eventually, the ride ends. For some, it ends with a joyful discharge—the car seat is finally buckled, and the hospital doors open to the fresh air of a new life. For others, it ends with a bittersweet goodbye, where the car seat stays empty, but the heart is overflowing with a love that embodies a lifetime. And for some, the ride leads to the long road of continued care, where home looks a little different but no less sacred.

However your ride ends, know this: You will survive it. You already are. You are not just waiting for the journey; you are being forged by it. Every time you show up, every time you whisper through the glass, and every time you choose hope over fear, you are winning. You are stronger than the ride, you are deeper than the drops, and you are the steady heartbeat your baby relies on. Take a breath, Protector. *You are doing a beautiful job, and you are never walking this track alone.*

NOTES

I invite you to take a moment to write your heart steady, anchor your mind, and claim the peace that belongs to you in this very moment.

CHAPTER 6

A Letter to the One Carrying a Miracle in Their Heart

Healing is not about forgetting the storm or pretending it did not happen. It is about learning to stand on the shore again and realizing that even after the waves, you are still here and you are still whole.

The following pages are dedicated to a specific part of the NICU story—the journey of those whose babies did not make it home. This chapter is for the parents who have had to say goodbye to their baby far sooner than they ever imagined.

If you are currently in the middle of your own climb and your heart needs to stay focused only on the path directly in front of you, please know that **this chapter is optional**. You are the guardian of your own emotions, if you are not ready to sit with this part of the landscape, it is okay to turn the page and move forward to the next chapter.

However, if you are seeking to understand the depth of every story written in these rooms, or if you are the parent who is currently carrying a heart full of memories, these words are for you. I included this section because every life that touches this unit—no matter how brief—is a miracle that spoke without words.

Remember, whether you choose to read this now or save it for later, you are in a safe space. There is no right or wrong way to navigate this journey—there is only the path that leads you toward peace.

Dear Parent of an Angel,

I honor you as you find yourself in this transition today, there are moments in life that carry a weight words simply were not designed to hold. As a nurse who has walked these halls for many years, I have seen the profound strength it takes to navigate the space you are in right now. I do not presume to know the depth of your specific walk, but I do understand that you have just completed a journey of immense sacrificial love.

To the one who stood watch when the world felt like it was spinning out of control.

You are the Warrior's Warrior. You were the anchor in a reality that was steadily unraveling, the silent strength behind every breath, and the steady hand in the dark.

There is a truth I hope you can hold on to today—*you did not fail*. While the hum of the machines and the constant glow of monitors have faded into the background, nothing can change the fact that you were the only home your baby knew. Long before they were introduced to a clinical world, they understood the rhythm of your heart. They knew the vibration of your voice, the very first sound that made your baby feel safe.

While your *Pit Crew* worked tirelessly to manage the technical complexities of your baby's care, your baby was focused entirely on the warmth of your presence. To your baby, you were the sun in their life. Whether it was measured in minutes, days, or months, they never knew a second without being enveloped in your love. That kind of connection does not just pass through, it touches your bones. It changes the very marrow of who you are.

Your baby's strength has woven itself into your own resilience, becoming a permanent part of the person you are still becoming. The journey ahead may feel uncertain, and the light may feel a bit dimmer for a while, but please know that your baby's life was not a tragedy; it *is* a legacy of pure, unshakable light that now lives within the quiet spaces of your heart.

I want you to know that although the winter feels long, your smile will come again. There will be a day when you begin to feel the warmth of hope returning to your soul not as a replacement for what was but as a testament to the love that remains. You are not shattered. You are not broken. You are whole, even if it doesn't feel like it right now.

You gave everything your beautiful baby could ever hope for—a life defined entirely by being loved. You were their whole world, and you were exactly what they needed. For now, allow yourself the grace to just be. Your healing begins with that single soft exhale.

With deepest respect,

A nurse who stood in the quiet of the room, and a heart that will always honor your strength.

NOTES

I invite you to take a moment to write your heart steady, anchor your mind, and claim the peace that belongs to you in this very moment.

CHAPTER 7

Sustaining the Parent Behind the Miracle

To care for the life that began in the NICU, you must first honor the life that carries them through it.

Your healing is the foundation upon which your baby's future is built. We often think of the parent as the supporter of the little patient we are caring for. But in this unit, the parent is a form of life-support.

You cannot pour from an empty cup, and in the NICU, your cup is not just for you—it is the reservoir your baby drinks from. When you sustain yourself, you are fortifying your miracle. Your baby does not need a perfect parent; they need a present one. By anchoring your own heart, you ensure that your foundation remains unshakable. No matter how long the climb, you cannot be a steady anchor in a storm if you are drifting away yourself.

Just as we triage patients in the unit, you are encouraged to triage your own needs so your light does not dim. If you lose power, your baby loses their anchor. *Fueling yourself is not an act of indulgence; it is a tactical requirement for your baby's recovery*. So, when the NICU Paradox begins to pull you under, apply these three layers of sustainment:

1. **Protect your battery:** Your physical presence is a biological signal of safety for your baby. To provide that signal, you need rest, hydration, and movement. Taking an hour away from the bedside to breathe fresh air is not *leaving* your baby—it is *recharging* the anchor.

2. **Filter the Noise:** In the foggy midground, you may be bombarded with data, opinions, and your own intrusive should-haves. But, give yourself permission to silence the noise. You do not owe the world an update; you owe your baby your presence.

3. **Honor the *And*:** Overwhelm happens when we fight our feelings. This is an invitation to accept that you can feel exhausted *and* grateful. You can feel heartbroken *and* determined. By allowing these emotions to coexist, you stop wasting energy trying to *fix* how you feel and start using that energy to simply *be*.

The Invisible Vital Sign

While we are surrounded by monitors that track every breath and every heartbeat, there is no machine that can track the weight on a parent's soul. The blinking lights tell us about your baby's journey but stay silent about yours.

I want you to pause here and acknowledge the heavy, invisible load you are carrying. It is a weight that does not show up on a chart, yet it affects every move you make as a Protector. Because we cannot see it on a screen, it is easy to treat your own well-being like a luxury—something you will get to *if* there's time. But the truth is, *caring for your heart is healthcare.*

Just as we prioritize your baby's vitals, we must prioritize yours, because you are the most important part of your baby's environment.

Think of your emotional health as your ***Internal Weather***. Some days, the sky is clear, and you feel a surge of strength and fortitude. On other days, a sudden storm rolls in—anxiety makes your chest feel tight, or a heavy fog of sadness makes it hard to see the next step.

Seeking help to navigate this weather is not a sign that you are not enough; it is a sign that you are a leader who knows when to call in reinforcements. Whether it is a trusted friend, counselor, or a support group, reaching out ensures you stay strong as the anchor. If you have a physical injury, you may need physical therapy to strengthen your body to allow you to keep showing up. Tending to your heart is no different; it is **Physical Therapy for the Soul**. It is the way you reinforce your foundation, ensuring that no matter what the monitors say, you remain steady and strong.

Sustaining the Soul

Beyond the emotional weather, there are daily pillars of health that keep you standing. Throughout this journey, we have focused intently on your baby's nutrition, their sleep, and their growth. But as you move through this phase, that focus must gently expand to include you. Your body and mind have been in a state of *high alert*—a survival mode that served you well in the crisis—but now it is time to shift toward a pace you can sustain for the long road ahead.

Fueling the Anchor

Your brain needs real fuel to manage the unique stress of this transition. Since your body is the primary vehicle for your baby's advocacy, and like any high-performance system, it requires real fuel to manage the unique stress of this transition. While quick sugar offers a temporary lift, that energy is often short-lived. In the NICU, you need a steady burn rather than a flicker. Choosing stabilized fuel ensures you don't find yourself running on empty when your baby needs you the most. Below is a table that acts as a reference guide to stabilize your energy.

Your Energy Stabilization Reference Guide

Fuel Type	The Goal	Examples
High-Efficiency Proteins	The building blocks of your patience and focus.	Examples of high-efficiency proteins are greek yogurt, hard boiled eggs, almonds, or lean deli turkey
Complex Carbohydrates	These offer slow-release energy to get you through the ebbs.	Complex carbohydrates include whole-grain crackers, oatmeal, or a piece of whole fruit with the skin.
Hydration (The Gold Standard)	Hydration is your primary cognitive tool; dehydration can mimic anxiety.	Structured water, herbal teas (mothers, be sure to consult with your lactation nurse regarding these), or water with a pinch of sea salt are examples of ways to stay hydrated..
Strategic Healthy Fats	These are brain fuel for you as you make high-stakes decisions for your baby.	Included in healthy fats are avocado, walnuts, or a small square of dark chocolate.

The Micro-Fueling Strategy

You may not have thirty minutes for a meal, but you always have thirty-seconds for a micro-fuel. This approach allows you to integrate your well-being into the natural rhythm of your day, ensuring your nutrition is as responsive as the care being provided at the bedside. Instead of waiting for the perfect time to step away, you are proactively fueling your engine in manageable increments to maintain your fortitude.

The 3-Hour Check: Every three hours, perform a self-triage. Ask yourself: "Am I running on adrenaline or actual fuel?" If the answer is adrenaline, it is time for a high-efficiency protein or a complex carb to reset your baseline.

The Hydration Rule: Dehydration is a silent drain on your fortitude; it mimics symptoms of anxiety and physical exhaustion. To ensure you are meeting the goal of at least eight glasses of water a day, do not wait for a formal clinical update to reach for your bottle. Instead, tie your hydration to the consistent rhythms of the bedside, e.g, use care times (the times your baby is fed, assessed, or changed) to drink a full glass of water or take intentional sips of water when your *Pit Crew* checks on your baby, which could be several times in an hour.

Rest

Rest in the NICU is often interrupted by the sharp sound of alarms, and sleep at home can be haunted by *phantom beeps*. Even if you cannot get a full night's sleep, *aim for restorative sleep*—intentional windows where you dim the lights and put the phone away, allowing your nervous system to step down from the ledge of the roller coaster.

Reclaiming Your Physical Strength

In addition to fueling your body, we must talk about how you move it. When you are in the NICU, your body is often held in a state of rigid tension—shoulders hunched over an isolette (incubator), sitting stiff in hospital chairs, or standing for hours in a state of high alert. This physical stress stores itself in your muscles and nervous system. Try this reset posture to calm your muscles and nervous system.

The Purpose

To open your chest and signal to your nervous system that you are safe and in command. *Movement is not a luxury; it is a release.* This is not about training for a marathon; it is about gentle, intentional movement that tells your body it is safe to let go of the "fight-or-flight" response.

The Technique

Pull your shoulder blades back and down, as if you are trying to tuck them into your back pockets. Lift your chin slightly.

The Physical Reset

A ten-minute walk in the fresh air, some light stretching, or even just stepping outside to feel the sun on your face can lower your cortisol levels and clear the brain fog that comes with medical fatigue—this is a specific kind of exhaustion that goes far beyond just *feeling tired*.

It is the mental and emotional fog that comes from weeks or months of processing complex medical data, making high-stakes decisions, and living in a constant state of hyper-vigilance. It can make the simplest tasks feel impossible, a sign that your *Protector* battery is running dangerously low and needs to be recharged through rest and a change of scenery.

The Emotional Shift

Exercise is not only about changing how you look; it is also about changing how you feel. It increases endorphins—your body's built-in stress-fighter. They are chemicals released by your brain during physical activity or moments of joy that act like a natural 'reset button.' They help to dull the sharp edges of physical pain and create a sense of well-being, helping you move from a state of high-alert anxiety into a space of calm and focus.

Bonding as a Family

You and your partner may be on the same roller coaster, but you might be sitting in different seats. Carve out non-medical minutes—brief windows where you talk about anything *except* hospital stats, doctor's updates, or bills. If you are walking this path alone, carving out some *me-time* to focus on yourself can give you the strength you need to continue the journey. Use this time to reconnect with the people you were before this ride started—this is not selfish; this is survival.

To be a long-term anchor, you cannot live in a constant state of clinical emergency. These minutes of normalcy are the oxygen masks you put on yourselves so you have the fortitude to keep advocating for your baby.

If there are other children at home remember that they are looking to you for stability. Ten minutes of focused, one-on-one time where they are the center of your world can be more healing than an entire day of distracted presence. Protecting your bond with your partner and your other children is not taking away from your NICU baby; it is ensuring that the family they are coming home to is whole and strong. *Balance is survival, not perfection.*

Expanding the Circle of the Home

The heart of the home is not a building, and it is not defined by a traditional family tree. It is defined by the person who refuses to leave.

The Single Parent: You are carrying a double mantle of tenacity. In this room you are the sole anchor, the primary voice, and the entire world for your baby. There is a specific kind of bravery in being the only one to hear the midnight updates and the only one to hold onto hope. Please know that your resilience is not *half* of anything—it is a complete and heroic force because you are the only foundation; your own healing is not a luxury. It is the very thing that keeps your baby's world steady. We see you and applaud your efforts.

To the Adoptive Parent: Your journey to this bedside followed a different map, but your role as *home* is absolute. The connection you are forging here is not built on a clinical history; it is built on the soul-deep choice to be the one who stays. You are not a "substitute" or a "visitor"—you are the intended destination. The love you pour into the silence of this unit is the first and most important medicine your baby will ever receive.

Whether you are navigating this journey alone or through the sacred bond of adoption, the womb hug you provide is the same. Your presence is the gold standard of care. You are the heartbeat your baby is listening for, and you are exactly the home they need.

The Strength in Accepting Help

In the NICU, you become the ultimate guardian. You learn to manage the monitors, the schedules, and the high-stake decisions. Because of this, it can feel like you are the only one who can carry the weight. *Accepting help is not a sign that you are failing; it is the mark of a wise leader who knows how to manage their resources.*

When you allow someone else to protect you, you are protecting your baby. By letting a friend bring dinner, a neighbor do a load of laundry, or a family member watch the siblings at home, you are clearing the mental space you need to remain the "Living Anchor" for your baby.

The "*Yes*" of Survival: Every time you say "yes" to a helping hand, you are saying "no" to burnout. You are making sure the foundation of your family stays strong for the long climb.

Releasing the "Guilt-Debt": When someone offers to bring a meal, run an errand, or sit with your other children, your first instinct might be to calculate the cost. You might find yourself thinking, *If I let them do this now, how will I ever pay them back?* I would like to invite you to look at this through a different lens. For those who love you, watching you go through the NICU journey can be incredibly painful because there is so little they can fix. They cannot breathe for your baby, and they cannot take away the *G-force* of the roller coaster.

Their offer of help is not a transaction; it is their way of standing in the gap. When they bring that dinner or fold that laundry, they are not looking for a trade. They are not keeping a tally for the future. They are simply trying to find a tangible way to say, *"I see you, I love you, and I am here."* By saying yes, you are not creating a debt—you are giving them a gift of being able to support the people they care about the most.

Accepting help is an act *of Strategic Surrender.* It is choosing to let go of the "small things" so you have the strength to hold on to the "big things." You do not have to carry the whole world on your shoulders to be a good parent. You just have to be the heartbeat of your home, and sometimes, a heartbeat needs a little help to keep its rhythm.

Knowing Your Limits

Part of accepting help is being honest about where your "ledge" is. In the NICU, you are often living on a high-stakes precipice, balancing medical data, family needs, and your own survival. Acknowledging that you are standing too close to the ledge isn't an admission of defeat; it is an act of extreme self-awareness.

You do not have to be a "super-parent" every hour of every day. In fact, trying to white-knuckle it while standing on that ledge is how medical fatigue turns into a permanent, dangerous fog. Acknowledging when you have hit your limit is an act of love. It tells your partner, your family, and your medical team exactly what you need to keep going. Whether it's needing an hour of silence, a night of sleep, or a professional to talk to, *knowing your limits is your superpower.* It ensures that when you *are* present, you aren't just a shadow of yourself —you are the vibrant, steady Protector your baby knows and loves.

You are already doing the impossible. You have whispered through an isolette (incubator), anchored a miracle, and fought for a legacy. Now take a breath. Look in the mirror and see what I see—a resilient, powerful soul who has built a life of love from the ground up.

You are worth the same care, the same patience, and the same deep love you so freely give to your baby. You are exactly where you need to be.

Now breathe and nourish your heart, recognizing that every breath you take and every ounce of strength you reclaim is a direct investment in the miracle your baby is fighting to achieve.

NOTES

I invite you to take a moment to write your heart steady, anchor your mind, and claim the peace that belongs to you in this very moment.

CHAPTER 8

Taking the Reigns

This is the moment the Pit Crew lets go and you take over, stepping into your true power as the heart, the soul, and forever guardian of your baby's story.

For a long time, your heart was beating to a rhythm that was not entirely your own. You have lived in a world where time was measured by the quiet unfolding of a new strength, and progress was counted in the steady, deepening peace of a sleeping baby. You have navigated a landscape where hope was a fragile life, held together by the glow of a screen and the hum of a room that never truly sleeps. You had a bedside vigil.

Even as you prepare to leave, you might feel the phantom pull of the unit—that sudden urge to check a pulse that is no longer wired to a sensor or the way your breath catches at the sound that mimics a hospital alarm.

This is the emotional ebb and flow of a soul that has been in a storm for too long. It is natural to feel a strange mix of soaring relief and a heavy, quiet trembling. You are stepping off a high-speed rollercoaster and onto solid ground, and it takes time for your equilibrium to return. Be patient with your heart as it learns the pace of a world without sirens—a world where time is finally measured in the soft weight of your baby in your arms, the steady rhythm of a rocking chair, and the peaceful, unhurried stillness of your own home.

The Sacred Handover

As the double doors of the unit close behind you for the final time, you are not just leaving a building; you are concluding a deep, complex partnership. Your *Pit Crew* have been silent witnesses to your most fragile moments. They held the space for your baby when your own arms were not available to do so. It is a sacred moment when the team steps back and the lead role returns fully to you.

Find comfort in knowing that the bond you built with your care team is a lasting foundation. You are not losing your safety net; you are graduating into independence, carrying their belief in you back to your front door.

You are leaving as the sovereign *Protector* of your baby, equipped with a strength that was forged behind hospital walls. Closing this circle allows you to walk forward with peace, knowing you were never alone in the fight, and you are not alone now—you have everything you need.

Your Home Toolkit

Stepping over your home threshold is the victory you hoped and prayed for, but it often brings a new kind of shadow of what-ifs. Knowledge is the only thing that can quiet the noise of a mind that has been on high alert for too long. These resources are here to help you with your transition home.

The Emergency Brake: Think of infant safety as your final piece of armor.

Cardiopulmonary Resuscitation (CPR): Taking a course is not about expecting a crisis; it is about having the skills to steady the track if it gets bumpy. It is the peace of mind that allows you to look at your baby's face instead of just watching their chest rise and fall.

Safe Sleep: In the NICU, your baby is often positioned for medical necessity, but at home you are the guardian of their sleep environment. Following safe sleep guidelines—placing your baby on their back, on a firm, flat surface free of blankets or toys—is how you maintain the womb hug in a way that is safe for the real world. These habits are the invisible guardrails that protect your baby while you finally allow yourself to rest.

The *When to Call* Protocol: To keep yourself from living on the ledge, work with your pediatrician to create a "maintenance list." Knowing exactly which symptoms require a phone call—and which ones are just the beautiful, messy signs of a baby growing—gives you the medical permission to breathe.

Trusting the Invisible Monitor: The physical screens stay behind, but you are taking your monitor of intuition home. You have survived the NICU, and you have been trained by the best. No machine can compete with the internal compass of a parent who has lived through this. If your gut says something is off, listen to it. You are the world's leading expert on your baby. Trusting your instincts is the highest form of healthcare.

Building Your Community

While you are leaving the unit, you are not leaving the strength of people you met there. There is a village of survivors waiting to embrace you and your family. Finding your community is how you turn your shared history into a future of support.

The Tribe of the Trenches: Those parents you nodded to in the hallway speak your language. It is ok to keep in touch with the ones you trust for NICU-safe playdates, where the boundaries of health and safety are already understood without explanation.

Digital Sanctuaries and Organizations: Look for moderated NICU support groups and organizations dedicated to post-discharge care. If your hospital does not have a group, ask your social worker about local or virtual options. Also, see the additional resources shared in *Appendix B – Unified Resources*.

Joining these groups is not about admitting you cannot cope alone; it is about accepting the specialized aftercare your family deserves.

A Gentle Compass for the Digital World

While the online world can be a beautiful sanctuary, remember to guard your heart as you navigate it. Not every story you read will be your story, and not every piece of advice is universal truth.

Your Team is the Gold Standard: Think of online groups as a place for emotional support but keep your pit crew as your source for medical truth. Always run new information by your care team—they have a unique map for your baby's journey.

Protect Your Peace: If a group or thread starts to feel like a weight rather than upliftment, give yourself the grace to walk away. If it increases anxiety rather than grounding your soul, it has served its purpose, and it is okay to leave. Your mental well-being is the atmosphere your baby breathes—keep it clear, kind, and focused on your own path.

Welcome Home

Eventually, the roller-coaster track levels out. The beeps quiet and fade into the background noise of a living, breathing home. Whether you walked out of these hospitals with a car seat, a baby with extra accessories, or a heart full of sacred, bittersweet memories, you have survived the impossible.

You are already doing it. You have anchored a miracle in the middle of the storm and fought for a legacy. You have learned to navigate the ledge and found the strength to ask for help when the climb got too steep. Remember: healing does not demand productivity. But for some, advocacy brings purpose from pain.

Now, I would like you to take a breath, look in the mirror, and say these words:

> *"I am more than a survivor. I am resilient, powerful, and wise. I am a steady light. I have built a foundation of love from the ground up, and it is unshakeable. I will carry the knowledge that I survived something most people cannot imagine."*

You are not alone. You never were. Thousands of parents have walked this path before you, and thousands walk it now beside you. Whether your child is in your arms or in your heart, they are so blessed to have you—and you are stronger than you will ever know.

Step into your healing and find your peace; you are finally home and on your way to being whole.

As we wave farewell from your NICU Pit Crew, our shift at your bedside comes to an end. The monitors quiet down, the lines are cleared, and a new journey is about to begin—but the truth of what was forged here remains permanent.

We have adjusted the machines, checked the vitals, and stood guard—but we were only ever the crew. **You** are the driver. **You** are the anchor. We hand the mission over to you now.

For some of you, packing up means loading a car seat for a long-awaited ride home. For others, it means gathering specialized equipment and learning a new rhythm of care at home. And for some of you, it means packing away tiny blankets and memoirs, walking out with empty arms but carrying a sacred legacy of love for a baby whose fight was brief but infinite.

No matter what you are carrying out of this room today, do not doubt the caliber of your spirit. We have watched you face the absolute limits of human endurance and still choose to own your strength. You may have come into this space terrified, but you are leaving it battle-tested, resilient, and deeply changed.

Remember always that you have everything you need inside you to walk through any weather that lies ahead, so go with the grace and power to honor your legacy.

NOTES

I invite you to take a moment to write your heart steady, anchor your mind, and claim the peace that belongs to you in this very moment.

Epilogue: A Parent's Heart

We have walked through the clinical steps, unpacked the medical terms, and learned how to navigate the complex realities of your baby's care. Throughout this journey, my hope has been to stand beside you, helping you find your footing in this tender, overwhelming world. But as we reach the end of this book, I would like us to step away from the monitors and the medicine. Allow me to sit beside you, parent to parent, and share a heart-to-heart moment.

If you close this book and look at the front cover, your eyes will see a picture of a tiny foot. That foot belongs to one of my own children.

Full disclosure: *none of my children were ever in the NICU.* They have never slept under phototherapy lights; they were never tethered to machines that beep in the dark, quiet moments. However, I do not need a medical chart to understand the quiet terror of parental uncertainty. I deeply recognize that fragile space you find yourself in when your baby is unwell, and a wave of absolute helplessness hits you. I hold space for the feeling of looking at your baby and realizing that, in this moment, there is nothing your hands can physically do to fix them.

In those heavy hours, the deepest instinct of a parent is *to protect.* We would willingly, without a second thought, take their place. We would absorb every ounce of their pain and carry the entire weight of their illness on our own shoulders just so they would not have to.

But parenthood brings us face-to-face with a beautiful yet heartbreaking truth: *we cannot.*

There are some journeys our children must walk on their own. Their tiny bodies must fight their own battles, find their own strength, and take their own steps. We cannot walk the path for them; we can only stand lovingly by their side, holding their hand through it all.

I honor that your family's journey is entirely unique. Your fears, your milestones, and your days will not look like anyone else's. But the heart of a parent is a universal language. There is a love we hold for our children, a quiet closeness no medicine can measure.

My hope is for you to know that this book has been wrapped in the deep empathy of a parent who comprehends the weight you are carrying. What closer, gentler way to show that connection than by sharing the image of a child I held inside my womb and close to my heart. That tiny foot on the cover is my way of reminding you that our parental hearts hold this connection of love.

You have faced the long clinical days and survived the heaviest moments of this season. As you close this final page, take a deep breath. Look at your beautiful baby--whether they are resting safely in your arms tonight, or whether they left this world too soon, leaving a space that can never be filled.

To the parents whose babies did not make it home, please know your journey is not forgotten. Your baby's footsteps were brief, but they left an indelible mark on this world, and the love you poured into them remains infinite.

To every parent reading this: *your love is the safest, most sacred place for your child's soul, and you are never walking this path alone.*

Appendix A

The Language of the Pit Crew (Medical Glossary)

Apnea: When pauses occur in your baby's breathing lasting more than 20 seconds at a time.

Adjusted Age: The age your baby would be if they had been born on their actual due date.

Bilirubin: The substance that causes jaundice when levels in the blood get too high after your baby is born. This can be treated with phototherapy.

Bradycardia (Brady): This is when the heart rate slows down and is sometimes accompanied by apnea.

Continuous Positive Airway Pressure (CPAP): This is a steady stream of air that helps keep your baby's lungs open and supported, making it easier for them to breathe on their own as they grow stronger.

Desaturation (Desat): This is the sudden or gradual decrease in your baby's oxygen level.

Gavage Feeding: This is a way to provide vital nutrition to your baby through a small, soft tube to the stomach. This ensures your baby gets the fuel they need to grow while still learning to eat on their own.

Intubation: When a small, flexible breathing tube is placed into your baby's airway to help your baby breathe. This ensures your baby receives precise support their body needs to rest and heal.

Isolette: This is an enclosed incubator providing warmth and protection for your baby.

Jaundice: This is the yellowing of your baby's skin and/or eyes from elevated bilirubin levels.

Kangaroo Care: This is the skin-to-skin contact between you and your baby.

Necrotizing Enterocolitis (NEC): This is a serious intestinal condition in which intestinal tissue becomes inflamed, requiring your Pit Crew to pause feedings and focus all medical efforts on healing your baby's digestive system.

Nasogastric (NG) Tube: This is a soft, flexible tube used for feeding your baby. It goes through your baby's nose to their stomach.

Neonatal Intensive Care Unit (NICU): This is a specialized environment where dedicated experts provide round-the-clock medical care and advanced support to help your baby grow, heal, and thrive. Some babies may need NICU stays up to six months of life. If your baby feels unwell after discharge and needs medical care, it is encouraged that they be taken to an Emergency Room for further assessment.

Phototherapy: This is a special light treatment for jaundice, which acts as a helper to get rid of excess bilirubin so your baby's body stays in a balanced state.

Pulse Oximeter: This is a device that monitors the oxygen saturation level of your baby.

Respiratory Distress: This is when your baby has difficulty breathing.

Ventilator: This machine helps your baby to breathe.

Appendix B

Unified Resources - Directory for the Warrior's Warrior

NATIONAL RESOURCES

Graham's Foundation

To deliver practical tools and care packages that help you manage the day-to-day stress of the bedside vigil and stay focused on your child's progress.

Website: grahamsfoundation.org

Contact: 1-888-466-2948

Liaison: Trained parent mentors

Hand to Hold

A community that pairs you with another parent mentor who has already survived the NICU journey, ensuring you have a personal guide to help you navigate the emotional climb and the transition back home.

Website: handtohold.org

Contact: 1-855-422-6428

Liaison: Family Support Navigators and peer mentors

Little Giraffe Foundation

To make the NICU feel less like a facility and more like a home by funding neonatal medical research and providing grants that help families bridge the gap between the hospital and their household.

Website: littlegiraffefoundation.org

Liaison: NICU Social Workers and Child Life Specialists (who often manage their support grants)

March of Dimes

To fight for the health of every mother and child, ensuring that no matter the circumstances of your birth story, you have the research and advocacy needed to thrive.

Website: marchofdimes.org

Contact: 1888-MODIMES (1-888-663-4637)

Liaison: On-site Family Support Coordinators (available in many NICUs -ask your social worker)

Project Sweet Peas

To provide small comforts and financial lifelines that allow you to focus on being the heart and soul of your child's care.

Website: projectsweetpeas.com

Liaison: Regional Leads for care package coordination

HELPFUL RESOURCES FOR PARENTS EXPERIENCING INFANT LOSS

International Stillbirth Alliance (ISA)

To unite voices across the globe to prevent loss and to ensure that every parent who says goodbye is treated with the highest level of respect and dignity.

Website: stillbirthalliance.org

Liaison: International Bereavement Advocacy groups

Rachel's Gift

To provide compassionate guidance and support for families who experience pregnancy or infant loss, ensuring that no parent walks through the journey of loss alone.

Website: rachelsgift.org

Contact: 1-404-545-4254

Liaison: Bereavement Doulas and support specialists

Share Pregnancy & Infant Loss Support

To bridge the gap between hospital and home for grieving parents, offering a lifelong network of groups and resources that honor the weight of your baby's story.

Website: nationalshare.org

Contact: 1-800-821-6819

Liaison: Support group coordinators

GLOBAL RESOURCES

European Foundation for the Care of Newborn Infants (EFCNI)

To set a global standard for newborn care, advocating for parents to be treated as essential partners - not visitors- in hospitals worldwide.

Website: efcni.org

Liaison: Parent organization network leads

Global Alliance for Newborn Care (GLANCE)

To give a worldwide voice to NICU families, focusing on making medical care respectful of the culture and specific needs of every family, everywhere.

Website: glance-network.org

Liaison: Global advocacy representatives

Post Partum Support International (PSI)

To protect the mental health of the parent, offering specialized online meetings that address the unique trauma and exhaustion associated with the intensive care journey.

Website: postpartum.net

Contact: 1-800-944-4773 (Text or Call)

Liaison: Specialized NICU support group facilitators

Additional Resources from Melecia

Wrap Yourself In Some Loving Support

You purchased this book to support your healing through this tumultuous time in your, and your baby's life. I have shared invaluable resources within these pages, and also offer them as downloadable files that you can print off, and have as reminders.

Visit my website: meleciaharriottmorant.com

Select the **Resources Page** and explore the resources that are available for you.

Feel free to share any of these resources with other parents who may need them and remind them that they are never alone on this journey.

With love and gratitude always.

Melecia Harriott-Morant

www.ingramcontent.com/pod-product-compliance
Lightning Source LLC
LaVergne TN
LVHW051923051126
851857LV00021B/2115
* 9 7 9 8 9 9 6 3 6 4 3 7 4 *